GASTROPARESIS DIET COOKBOOK

The Ultimate Soothing Diet Recipes to Relief Gastroparesis

Joel Thompson

CONTENTS

Title Page

Copyright

Introduction

CHAPTER ONE   1

CHAPTER TWO   4

CHAPTER THREE   23

CHAPTER FOUR   42

CHAPTER FIVE   64

CHAPTER SIX   78

CHAPTER SEVEN   94

Conclusion   100

INTRODUCTION

Explanation of Gastroparesis and How It Affects Digestion

Gastroparesis is a medical condition in which the stomach muscles are damaged or weakened, leading to slow or incomplete digestion of food. The condition can affect anyone, but it is more common in women than men, and it is most commonly found in people who have diabetes. The cause of gastroparesis is not always known, but it can be related to nerve damage or an underlying autoimmune disorder.

When food is not properly digested in the stomach, it can cause a range of uncomfortable symptoms. The most common symptoms of gastroparesis include nausea, vomiting, abdominal pain or discomfort, bloating, and a feeling of fullness after eating only a small amount of food. People with gastroparesis may also experience weight loss, malnutrition, and dehydration due to their inability to properly digest and absorb nutrients from their food.

There is no cure for gastroparesis, but there are treatments that can help manage the symptoms. Medications such as prokinetic drugs can help stimulate the muscles in the stomach and promote more regular digestion. Changes to the diet, such as eating smaller meals more frequently and avoiding foods that are difficult to digest, can also be helpful in managing symptoms.

Overview of the Gastroparesis Diet and Why It's Important

The gastroparesis diet is a specific eating plan designed to help people with gastroparesis manage their symptoms and improve their overall digestive health. The diet focuses on eating smaller, more frequent meals throughout the day, and avoiding foods that are difficult to digest or that can exacerbate gastroparesis symptoms.

Some of the key dietary changes that are recommended for people with gastroparesis include:

- Eating smaller, more frequent meals: This can help ease the workload on the stomach and make digestion easier.

- Avoiding high-fat foods: Fatty foods can slow down digestion and make gastroparesis symptoms worse.

- Avoiding high-fiber foods: Fibrous foods can be difficult to digest and can cause bloating, cramping, and other digestive issues.

- Choosing softer, more easily digestible foods: Foods that are soft and easy to chew and swallow, such as cooked vegetables, lean protein, and whole grains, are typically recommended for people with gastroparesis.

- Drinking plenty of fluids: Staying hydrated is important for overall digestive health and can help alleviate some gastroparesis symptoms.

Following a gastroparesis diet can be challenging, but it can also be extremely helpful in managing symptoms and improving overall quality of life for people with the condition.

Explanation of How the Cookbook Can Help Those with Gastroparesis

Cookbooks specifically designed for people with gastroparesis can be an incredibly helpful resource for those living with the condition. These cookbooks offer a range of recipes that are tailored to the unique dietary needs and restrictions of people with gastroparesis, making it easier to plan and prepare meals that are both nutritious and easy to digest.

Some of the key benefits of using a gastroparesis cookbook include:

- Access to a wide range of recipe ideas: A gastroparesis cookbook can offer a wealth of recipe ideas that are specifically designed for people with the condition, making it easier to plan meals and try new dishes.

- Tailored to specific dietary needs: A gastroparesis cookbook can help take the guesswork out of meal planning by offering recipes that are tailored to the unique dietary needs and restrictions of people with gastroparesis.

- Offers helpful tips and strategies: Many gastroparesis cookbooks also include tips and strategies for managing symptoms, such as ideas for portion control, ways to incorporate more nutrient-dense foods into the diet, and tips for staying hydrated.

- Can provide inspiration and motivation: Trying to manage gastroparesis symptoms through diet can be challenging, and it can be easy to fall into a rut of eating the same foods over and over again. A gastroparesis cookbook can provide inspiration and motivation to try new recipes and experiment with different flavors and ingredients.

When using a gastroparesis cookbook, it's important to remember that not all recipes will work for everyone. People with gastroparesis may have different tolerances for certain foods, and it's important to listen to your body and adjust recipes as needed. It's also a good idea to consult with a healthcare provider or registered dietitian before making any significant changes to your diet.

In addition to using a gastroparesis cookbook, there are other strategies that can help manage symptoms and improve digestive health. These may include medications to stimulate stomach contractions, changes in eating habits such as eating smaller, more frequent meals, and avoiding foods that exacerbate symptoms. Working with a healthcare provider or registered dietitian can help identify the best strategies for managing gastroparesis symptoms and improving overall digestive health.

CHAPTER ONE

Gastroparesis Diet Basics

Overview of the Gastroparesis Diet

Gastroparesis is a digestive disorder that affects the stomach's ability to empty food at a normal rate. People with gastroparesis may experience symptoms such as nausea, vomiting, abdominal pain, and bloating. While there is no cure for gastroparesis, changes to diet and lifestyle can help manage symptoms.

The primary goal of a gastroparesis diet is to reduce symptoms and ensure that the body is getting the necessary nutrients. This typically involves eating smaller, more frequent meals and avoiding foods that are difficult to digest. A dietitian can help create an individualized plan that takes into account a person's specific symptoms and nutritional needs.

List of Foods to Avoid

Certain foods can be difficult to digest and should be avoided or limited in a gastroparesis diet. Some examples include:

1. High-fat foods: Foods high in fat can slow down the digestive process and exacerbate symptoms of gastroparesis. This includes fried foods, fatty cuts of meat, and full-fat dairy products.

2. Fibrous foods: Foods high in fiber, such as raw

vegetables, whole grains, and nuts, can be difficult to digest and may worsen symptoms.

3. Carbonated beverages: Carbonation can increase feelings of bloating and discomfort in people with gastroparesis.

4. Alcohol: Alcohol can slow down the digestive process and may lead to nausea and vomiting.

5. Spicy foods: Spicy foods can irritate the stomach lining and exacerbate symptoms of gastroparesis.

6. Large meals: Eating large meals can overwhelm the stomach and make symptoms worse. It is recommended to eat smaller, more frequent meals throughout the day.

List of Recommended Foods

While there are certain foods to avoid with gastroparesis, there are also foods that can help manage symptoms and provide important nutrients. Here are some examples:

1. Low-fat foods: Foods that are low in fat are easier to digest and less likely to worsen symptoms. Some examples include lean cuts of meat, low-fat dairy products, and tofu.

2. Soft, cooked vegetables: Vegetables that are soft and cooked are easier to digest than raw vegetables. Some examples include steamed carrots, squash, and sweet potatoes.

3. Soups and broths: Soups and broths can be a good source of nutrients and are easier to digest than solid foods.

4. Low-fiber fruits: Fruits that are low in fiber, such as bananas, melons, and peaches, are easier to

digest and less likely to exacerbate symptoms.

5. Grains and cereals: Grains and cereals that are low in fiber, such as white rice, pasta, and oatmeal, can be a good source of carbohydrates and are easier to digest than whole grains.

6. Small, frequent meals: Eating smaller, more frequent meals throughout the day can help manage symptoms and ensure that the body is getting the necessary nutrients.

In conclusion, while there is no cure for gastroparesis, changes to diet and lifestyle can help manage symptoms. Avoiding difficult-to-digest foods and eating smaller, more frequent meals can be helpful. It is also important to work with a dietitian to create an individualized plan that takes into account a person's specific symptoms and nutritional needs.

CHAPTER TWO

Breakfast Recipes

Easy-to-digest breakfast recipes

Banana Oatmeal Pancakes

These pancakes are a delicious and healthy way to start your day. They're made with whole grain oats and ripe bananas, which provide natural sweetness and a boost of potassium. The texture is fluffy and satisfying, making them a great breakfast option for the whole family.

Ingredients:

- 1 cup old-fashioned oats
- 1 ripe banana
- 1 egg
- 1/4 cup almond milk
- 1 tsp baking powder
- 1/2 tsp vanilla extract
- Pinch of salt
- Cooking spray

Instructions:

1. In a blender or food processor, blend oats until they form a fine powder.
2. Add banana, egg, almond milk, baking powder, vanilla extract, and salt to the blender. Blend until

smooth.

3. Heat a non-stick skillet over medium heat. Spray with cooking spray.

4. Pour pancake batter onto the skillet, using about 1/4 cup for each pancake.

5. Cook until bubbles form on the surface and the edges begin to dry, about 2-3 minutes.

6. Flip the pancake and cook for an additional minute.

7. Serve warm with your favorite toppings, such as sliced bananas, berries, or maple syrup.

Nutritional Information:

- Calories: 327
- Protein: 13g
- Fat: 7g
- Carbohydrates: 57g
- Fiber: 9g

Scrambled Tofu

This vegan breakfast option is a high-protein alternative to scrambled eggs. Tofu is crumbled and seasoned with a blend of spices and vegetables, creating a flavorful and satisfying dish that's perfect for any time of day.

Ingredients:

- 1 block of firm tofu
- 1/2 onion, diced
- 1/2 red bell pepper, diced
- 1 clove garlic, minced
- 1 tbsp olive oil

- 1 tsp turmeric
- 1/2 tsp cumin
- 1/4 tsp paprika
- Salt and pepper to taste

Instructions:

1. Drain the tofu and crumble it with a fork.
2. In a large skillet, heat olive oil over medium heat.
3. Add onion and bell pepper to the skillet and cook until softened, about 5 minutes.
4. Add garlic and spices to the skillet and cook for an additional 2 minutes.
5. Add crumbled tofu to the skillet and cook for 5-7 minutes, stirring occasionally.
6. Serve hot with toast or tortillas.

Nutritional Information:

- Calories: 239
- Protein: 18g
- Fat: 16g
- Carbohydrates: 8g
- Fiber: 2g

Yogurt Parfait with Berries and Granola

This colorful and nutritious breakfast parfait is made with layers of creamy Greek yogurt, fresh berries, and crunchy granola. It's a great way to start your day with a balanced combination of protein, fiber, and antioxidants.

Ingredients:

- 1 cup Greek yogurt

- 1/2 cup mixed berries (such as strawberries, blueberries, and raspberries)
- 1/4 cup granola

Instructions:

1. In a glass or jar, add a layer of Greek yogurt.
2. Add a layer of mixed berries on top of the yogurt.
3. Sprinkle a layer of granola on top of the berries.
4. Repeat the layers until you reach the top of the glass.
5. Serve cold and enjoy!

Nutritional Information (per serving):

- Calories: 242
- Protein: 20g
- Fat: 7g
- Carbohydrates: 26g
- Fiber: 3g

Almond Butter and Banana Toast

This simple and delicious breakfast option is a great way to satisfy your cravings for something sweet and nutty. Whole grain toast is topped with creamy almond butter and ripe banana slices, creating a balanced and filling meal that's perfect for busy mornings.

Ingredients:

- 2 slices whole grain bread
- 2 tbsp almond butter
- 1 ripe banana, sliced

Instructions:

1. Toast the bread slices in a toaster or toaster oven until golden brown.
2. Spread almond butter evenly on each slice of toast.
3. Top each slice of toast with banana slices.
4. Serve warm and enjoy!

Nutritional Information:

- Calories: 375
- Protein: 13g
- Fat: 16g
- Carbohydrates: 50g
- Fiber: 9g

Smoothie recipes

Strawberry Banana Smoothie

This smoothie is a perfect blend of sweet and creamy, with a refreshing taste that will make you feel energized all day long. Made with fresh strawberries and ripe bananas, this smoothie is packed with essential nutrients that are good for your body.

Ingredients:

- 1 cup fresh strawberries, hulled and chopped
- 1 ripe banana, peeled and sliced
- 1/2 cup Greek yogurt
- 1/2 cup almond milk
- 1 tbsp honey
- 1/2 tsp vanilla extract
- Ice (optional)

Instructions:

1. In a blender, combine the chopped strawberries, sliced banana, Greek yogurt, almond milk, honey, and vanilla extract.

2. Blend the ingredients until smooth and creamy.

3. If you prefer a thicker smoothie, add some ice and blend again until well combined.

4. Pour the smoothie into a glass and enjoy.

Nutritional Information:

- Calories: 216 kcal
- Protein: 7 g
- Fat: 3 g
- Carbohydrates: 42 g
- Fiber: 4 g

Blueberry Spinach Smoothie

This smoothie is a healthy and refreshing way to start your day. It is packed with nutrients that will help boost your energy and keep you feeling full for longer. The combination of blueberries and spinach makes for a delicious and nutritious smoothie that you will want to enjoy every morning.

Ingredients:

- 1 cup fresh blueberries
- 1 cup fresh spinach
- 1/2 cup almond milk
- 1/2 cup Greek yogurt
- 1 tbsp honey

- 1/2 tsp vanilla extract
- Ice (optional)

Instructions:

1. In a blender, combine the blueberries, spinach, almond milk, Greek yogurt, honey, and vanilla extract.

2. Blend the ingredients until smooth and creamy.

3. If you prefer a thicker smoothie, add some ice and blend again until well combined.

4. Pour the smoothie into a glass and enjoy.

Nutritional Information:

- Calories: 192 kcal
- Protein: 9 g
- Fat: 3 g
- Carbohydrates: 34 g
- Fiber: 4 g

Peanut Butter Banana Smoothie

This smoothie is a delicious and healthy way to start your day. Made with peanut butter and banana, it is packed with protein and nutrients that will help keep you feeling full and satisfied. The combination of flavors in this smoothie is sure to please even the pickiest eaters.

Ingredients:

- 1 ripe banana, peeled and sliced
- 1/2 cup almond milk
- 1/2 cup Greek yogurt
- 1 tbsp peanut butter
- 1 tbsp honey

- 1/2 tsp vanilla extract
- Ice (optional)

Instructions:

1. In a blender, combine the sliced banana, almond milk, Greek yogurt, peanut butter, honey, and vanilla extract.

2. Blend the ingredients until smooth and creamy.

3. If you prefer a thicker smoothie, add some ice and blend again until well combined.

4. Pour the smoothie into a glass and enjoy.

Nutritional Information:

- Calories: 254 kcal
- Protein: 13 g
- Fat: 7 g
- Carbohydrates: 38 g
- Fiber: 4 g

Mango Pineapple Smoothie

This smoothie is a tropical delight, made with fresh mango and pineapple that will transport you to a beach in paradise. It is packed with essential nutrients and vitamins that will keep you feeling energized and healthy.

Ingredients:

- 1 cup fresh mango
- 1 cup fresh pineapple, chopped
- 1/2 cup Greek yogurt
- 1/2 cup almond milk

- 1 tbsp honey
- 1/2 tsp vanilla extract
- Ice (optional)

Instructions:

1. In a blender, combine the chopped mango, chopped pineapple, Greek yogurt, almond milk, honey, and vanilla extract.

2. Blend the ingredients until smooth and creamy.

3. If you prefer a thicker smoothie, add some ice and blend again until well combined.

4. Pour the smoothie into a glass and enjoy.

Nutritional Information:

- Calories: 218 kcal
- Protein: 7 g
- Fat: 3 g
- Carbohydrates: 41 g
- Fiber: 4 g

Oatmeal and porridge recipes

Apple Cinnamon Oatmeal

This Apple Cinnamon Oatmeal is the perfect breakfast for those who want something filling and warm to start their day. The combination of the sweet apples and cinnamon with the hearty oats will leave you feeling satisfied and ready to take on the day.

Ingredients:

- 1 cup rolled oats
- 2 cups water

- 1/2 teaspoon ground cinnamon
- 1/2 teaspoon vanilla extract
- 1 medium apple, diced
- 2 tablespoons maple syrup
- 1/4 cup chopped nuts (optional)

Instructions:

1. In a medium saucepan, combine the oats, water, cinnamon, and vanilla extract.

2. Bring to a boil over high heat, then reduce the heat to medium-low and simmer for 10-15 minutes, stirring occasionally, until the oats are tender and the mixture has thickened.

3. Stir in the diced apple and maple syrup and cook for an additional 2-3 minutes until the apple is heated through.

4. Serve hot, topped with chopped nuts if desired.

Nutritional Information:

- Calories: 300
- Fat: 7g
- Carbohydrates: 52g
- Fiber: 8g
- Protein: 8g

Coconut Milk Quinoa Porridge

This Coconut Milk Quinoa Porridge is a great alternative to traditional oatmeal, offering a nutty flavor and creamy texture. The coconut milk adds a touch of sweetness, while the quinoa provides a good source of protein to start your day off right.

Ingredients:

- 1 cup quinoa
- 2 cups water
- 1 cup coconut milk
- 1 tablespoon honey
- 1/2 teaspoon ground cinnamon
- 1/4 teaspoon salt
- 1/4 cup chopped nuts (optional)

Instructions:

1. Rinse the quinoa thoroughly in a fine mesh strainer and drain.
2. In a medium saucepan, combine the quinoa, water, coconut milk, honey, cinnamon, and salt.
3. Bring to a boil over high heat, then reduce the heat to medium-low and simmer for 15-20 minutes, stirring occasionally, until the quinoa is tender and the mixture has thickened.
4. Serve hot, topped with chopped nuts if desired.

Nutritional Information:

- Calories: 400
- Fat: 19g
- Carbohydrates: 49g
- Fiber: 5g
- Protein: 10g

Blueberry Buckwheat Porridge

This Blueberry Buckwheat Porridge is a gluten-free alternative to traditional oatmeal, offering a slightly nutty flavor and creamy texture. The blueberries add a sweet and tart flavor, while the buckwheat provides a good source of fiber and protein.

Ingredients:

- 1 cup buckwheat groats
- 2 cups water
- 1 cup almond milk
- 1/2 teaspoon ground cinnamon
- 1/4 teaspoon salt
- 1 cup fresh or frozen blueberries
- 2 tablespoons honey
- 1/4 cup chopped nuts (optional)

Instructions:

1. Rinse the buckwheat groats thoroughly in a fine mesh strainer and drain.

2. In a medium saucepan, combine the buckwheat groats, water, almond milk, cinnamon, and salt.

3. Bring to a boil over high heat, then reduce the heat to medium-low and simmer for 20-25 minutes, stirring occasionally, until the buckwheat is tender and the mixture has thickened.

4. Stir in the blueberries and honey and cook for an additional 2-3 minutes until the blueberries are heated through and the porridge has reached your desired consistency. 5. Serve hot, topped with chopped nuts if desired.

Nutritional Information:

- Calories: 350
- Fat: 8g
- Carbohydrates: 64g

- Fiber: 10g
- Protein: 9g

Chocolate Chia Seed Pudding

This Chocolate Chia Seed Pudding is a delicious and healthy dessert or breakfast option. The chia seeds provide a good source of fiber and omega-3 fatty acids, while the cocoa powder adds a rich and chocolatey flavor.

Ingredients:

- 1/2 cup chia seeds
- 2 cups almond milk
- 1/4 cup cocoa powder
- 1/4 cup honey or maple syrup
- 1 teaspoon vanilla extract
- 1/4 teaspoon salt
- Fresh fruit or chopped nuts for topping (optional)

Instructions:

1. In a medium bowl, whisk together the chia seeds, almond milk, cocoa powder, honey or maple syrup, vanilla extract, and salt until well combined.

2. Cover and refrigerate for at least 2 hours, or overnight, until the mixture has thickened into a pudding-like consistency.

3. Serve chilled, topped with fresh fruit or chopped nuts if desired.

Nutritional Information:

- Calories: 250
- Fat: 12g

- Carbohydrates: 30g
- Fiber: 13g
- Protein: 8g

Egg dishes

Veggie Omelette

Description: This veggie omelette is a delicious and healthy breakfast option that is perfect for those who want to start their day with a protein-packed meal. Loaded with colorful vegetables and savory cheese, this omelette is sure to satisfy your taste buds.

Ingredients:

- 2 large eggs
- 1/4 cup chopped bell pepper
- 1/4 cup chopped onion
- 1/4 cup chopped tomato
- 1/4 cup shredded cheddar cheese
- Salt and pepper to taste
- 1 tablespoon olive oil

Instructions:

1. In a small bowl, beat the eggs with a fork until well combined. Season with salt and pepper to taste.

2. Heat the olive oil in a non-stick skillet over medium-high heat.

3. Add the bell pepper, onion, and tomato to the skillet and sauté for 2-3 minutes until softened.

4. Pour the beaten eggs into the skillet and let cook for 1-2 minutes.

5. Sprinkle the shredded cheese on top of the eggs.

6. Use a spatula to fold the omelette in half and cook for another 1-2 minutes until the cheese is melted and the eggs are cooked to your liking.

7. Serve hot with your favorite breakfast sides.

Nutritional Information:

- Calories: 250
- Fat: 19g
- Protein: 15g
- Carbohydrates: 6g
- Fiber: 1g

Huevos Rancheros

Description: Huevos Rancheros is a traditional Mexican breakfast that is hearty, flavorful, and easy to make. This dish features fried eggs served on a bed of warm corn tortillas and topped with a zesty tomato sauce and fresh herbs.

Ingredients:

- 4 corn tortillas
- 4 large eggs
- 1/4 cup chopped onion
- 1/4 cup chopped bell pepper
- 1 garlic clove, minced
- 1/2 cup canned diced tomatoes
- 1/4 teaspoon chili powder
- Salt and pepper to taste
- 1 tablespoon olive oil
- Chopped cilantro for garnish

Instructions:

1. Heat the olive oil in a skillet over medium heat.

2. Add the onion, bell pepper, and garlic to the skillet and sauté for 2-3 minutes until softened.

3. Add the canned tomatoes and chili powder to the skillet and stir to combine. Simmer for 5-10 minutes until the sauce has thickened.

4. While the sauce is simmering, heat the tortillas in a separate skillet over medium heat until warm and slightly toasted.

5. Fry the eggs in a non-stick skillet to your desired doneness.

6. To assemble the dish, place a tortilla on a plate, top with a fried egg, and spoon the tomato sauce over the egg.

7. Garnish with chopped cilantro and serve hot.

Nutritional Information:

- Calories: 300
- Fat: 15g
- Protein: 12g
- Carbohydrates: 30g
- Fiber: 4g

Shakshuka

Description: Shakshuka is a classic Middle Eastern breakfast dish that is easy to make and full of flavor. This dish features eggs poached in a tomato-based sauce and seasoned with a variety of spices and fresh herbs.

Ingredients:

- 1 tablespoon olive oil
- 1 onion, diced
- 1 red bell pepper, diced
- 3 garlic cloves, minced
- 1 teaspoon paprika
- 1/2 teaspoon ground cumin
- 1/4 teaspoon cayenne pepper
- 1/4 teaspoon salt
- 1/4 teaspoon black pepper
- 1 can (14 oz) diced tomatoes
- 4-6 large eggs
- Chopped parsley or cilantro for garnish

Instructions:

1. Heat the olive oil in a large skillet over medium heat.

2. Add the diced onion and bell pepper and sauté for 5-7 minutes until softened.

3. Add the minced garlic and spices (paprika, cumin, cayenne pepper, salt, and black pepper) to the skillet and stir to combine.

4. Add the canned diced tomatoes to the skillet and bring the mixture to a simmer.

5. Use a spoon to make small wells in the tomato sauce and crack an egg into each well.

6. Cover the skillet and let the eggs poach in the sauce for 5-7 minutes until the whites are set but the yolks are still runny.

7. Garnish with chopped parsley or cilantro and

serve hot with crusty bread or pita.

Nutritional Information:

- Calories: 180
- Fat: 11g
- Protein: 11g
- Carbohydrates: 12g
- Fiber: 3g

Avocado Egg Salad

Description: Avocado egg salad is a delicious and healthy twist on classic egg salad. This recipe is made with ripe avocado, hard-boiled eggs, and a variety of fresh herbs and spices.

Ingredients:

- 4 hard-boiled eggs, peeled and chopped
- 1 ripe avocado, peeled and pitted
- 1/4 cup chopped onion
- 1/4 cup chopped celery
- 2 tablespoons plain Greek yogurt
- 1 tablespoon Dijon mustard
- 1 tablespoon chopped fresh cilantro or parsley
- Salt and pepper to taste

Instructions:

1. In a large bowl, mash the ripe avocado with a fork until smooth.
2. Add the chopped hard-boiled eggs, onion, celery, Greek yogurt, Dijon mustard, and chopped herbs to the bowl and stir to combine.
3. Season with salt and pepper to taste.

4. Serve the avocado egg salad on toast or in lettuce cups for a low-carb option.

Nutritional Information:

- Calories: 250
- Fat: 19g
- Protein: 13g
- Carbohydrates: 8g
- Fiber: 6g

CHAPTER THREE

Lunch Recipes

Light and easy-to-digest lunch recipes

Avocado Chicken Salad

This Avocado Chicken Salad is a healthy and delicious meal that is perfect for lunch or dinner. The meal is made with cooked chicken, diced avocado, diced red onion, and cherry tomatoes. The dressing is a simple mixture of olive oil, lemon juice, Dijon mustard, salt, and black pepper.

Ingredients:

- 2 cups cooked chicken, shredded
- 1 ripe avocado, diced
- 1/2 cup diced red onion
- 1 cup cherry tomatoes, halved
- 1/4 cup olive oil
- 2 tablespoons lemon juice
- 1 tablespoon Dijon mustard
- Salt and black pepper to taste

Instructions:

1. In a large bowl, combine the cooked chicken, diced avocado, diced red onion, and halved cherry tomatoes.

2. In a small bowl, whisk together the olive oil,

lemon juice, Dijon mustard, salt, and black pepper.

3. Pour the dressing over the chicken mixture and toss to combine.

4. Serve immediately or refrigerate until ready to serve.

Nutritional Information:

- Calories: 378
- Fat: 28g
- Carbohydrates: 11g
- Protein: 22g
- Sugar: 3g

Quinoa and Vegetable Stir-Fry

This Quinoa and Vegetable Stir-Fry is a healthy and tasty vegetarian meal that is easy to make. The meal is made with quinoa, a variety of vegetables such as carrots, bell peppers, and broccoli, and a flavorful sauce made with soy sauce, garlic, and ginger.

Ingredients:

- 1 cup quinoa
- 2 cups water
- 2 tablespoons olive oil
- 1 onion, chopped
- 2 carrots, chopped
- 1 red bell pepper, chopped
- 2 cups broccoli florets
- 3 cloves garlic, minced

- 1 tablespoon grated fresh ginger
- 1/4 cup soy sauce
- Salt and black pepper to taste

Instructions:

1. Rinse the quinoa and combine with the water in a medium saucepan. Bring to a boil, then reduce the heat to low and simmer for 15-20 minutes until the water is absorbed and the quinoa is tender.

2. In a large skillet, heat the olive oil over medium-high heat. Add the chopped onion, chopped carrots, and chopped red bell pepper. Cook for 5-7 minutes until the vegetables are tender.

3. Add the broccoli florets, minced garlic, and grated ginger to the skillet. Cook for an additional 5-7 minutes until the broccoli is tender.

4. Add the cooked quinoa to the skillet and stir to combine.

5. In a small bowl, whisk together the soy sauce, salt, and black pepper. Pour the sauce over the quinoa and vegetables and stir to combine.

6. Serve hot.

Nutritional Information:

- Calories: 295
- Fat: 9g
- Carbohydrates: 46g
- Protein: 10g
- Sugar: 6g

Turkey and Hummus Wrap

This Turkey and Hummus Wrap is a healthy and delicious meal that is perfect for lunch on-the-go. The meal is made with sliced turkey breast, hummus, sliced cucumber, and shredded lettuce, all wrapped up in a whole wheat tortilla.

Ingredients:

- 1 whole wheat tortilla
- 3 slices of turkey breast
- 2 tablespoons hummus
- 1/4 cup sliced cucumber
- 1/2 cup shredded lettuce

Instructions:

1. Lay the whole wheat tortilla flat on a plate or cutting board.
2. Spread the hummus evenly over the tortilla.
3. Place the sliced turkey breast on top of the hummus.
4. Add the sliced cucumber and shredded lettuce on top of the turkey.
5. Roll the tortilla tightly, tucking in the sides as you go.
6. Slice the wrap in half and serve.

Nutritional Information:

- Calories: 254
- Fat: 7g
- Carbohydrates: 26g
- Protein: 21g
- Sugar: 2g

Tuna and White Bean Salad

This Tuna and White Bean Salad is a healthy and filling meal that is perfect for lunch or dinner. The meal is made with canned tuna, canned white beans, cherry tomatoes, and a simple dressing made with olive oil, lemon juice, Dijon mustard, salt, and black pepper.

Ingredients:

- 2 cans of tuna, drained
- 1 can of white beans, drained and rinsed
- 1 cup cherry tomatoes, halved
- 2 tablespoons olive oil
- 2 tablespoons lemon juice
- 1 tablespoon Dijon mustard
- Salt and black pepper to taste

Instructions:

1. In a large bowl, combine the drained tuna, drained and rinsed white beans, and halved cherry tomatoes.

2. In a small bowl, whisk together the olive oil, lemon juice, Dijon mustard, salt, and black pepper.

3. Pour the dressing over the tuna and bean mixture and toss to combine.

4. Serve immediately or refrigerate until ready to serve.

Nutritional Information:

- Calories: 327
- Fat: 12g
- Carbohydrates: 22g
- Protein: 34g

- Sugar: 2g

Soup and stew recipes

Lentil Soup

This hearty and nutritious **lentil soup** is a perfect meal for a cold evening. It's packed with protein, fiber, and vitamins that will keep you satisfied and nourished.

Ingredients:

- 1 cup dried lentils, rinsed and drained
- 1 onion, chopped
- 2 carrots, peeled and diced
- 2 celery stalks, diced
- 3 garlic cloves, minced
- 4 cups vegetable broth
- 1 teaspoon ground cumin
- 1 teaspoon ground coriander
- 1/2 teaspoon smoked paprika
- 1 bay leaf
- 2 tablespoons olive oil
- Salt and pepper to taste

Instructions:

1. In a large pot, heat olive oil over medium heat. Add onion, carrots, celery, and garlic. Sauté for 5-7 minutes or until the vegetables are soft.

2. Add lentils, vegetable broth, cumin, coriander, smoked paprika, bay leaf, salt, and pepper. Stir well.

3. Bring the mixture to a boil, then reduce heat to

low and let it simmer for 30-40 minutes or until the lentils are tender.

4. Remove the bay leaf and serve hot.

Nutritional Information:

This lentil soup recipe makes 4 servings. Each serving contains approximately:

- 250 calories
- 15g protein
- 40g carbohydrates
- 5g fat
- 15g fiber

Chicken Noodle Soup

This classic **chicken noodle soup** recipe is a comfort food that's perfect for any time of the year. It's packed with tender chicken, hearty vegetables, and delicious noodles.

Ingredients:

- 2 chicken breasts, cooked and shredded
- 1 onion, chopped
- 3 garlic cloves, minced
- 2 celery stalks, diced
- 2 carrots, peeled and diced
- 6 cups chicken broth
- 2 cups egg noodles
- 1 tablespoon olive oil
- 1 teaspoon dried thyme
- Salt and pepper to taste

Instructions:

1. In a large pot, heat olive oil over medium heat. Add onion, garlic, celery, and carrots. Sauté for 5-7 minutes or until the vegetables are soft.

2. Add chicken broth, shredded chicken, thyme, salt, and pepper. Bring the mixture to a boil, then reduce heat to low and let it simmer for 15-20 minutes.

3. Add egg noodles and cook for an additional 10-12 minutes or until they're tender.

4. Serve hot.

Nutritional Information:

This chicken noodle soup recipe makes 6 servings. Each serving contains approximately:

- 250 calories
- 20g protein
- 20g carbohydrates
- 10g fat
- 2g fiber

Beef Stew

This **beef stew** recipe is a delicious and hearty meal that's perfect for a cozy night in. It's packed with tender beef, flavorful vegetables, and a rich broth that will warm you up from the inside out.

Ingredients:

- 2 lbs beef stew meat, cubed
- 1 onion, chopped
- 3 garlic cloves, minced
- 4 carrots, peeled and chopped

- 4 celery stalks, chopped
- 4 potatoes, peeled and chopped
- 4 cups beef broth
- 2 tablespoons tomato paste
- 1 tablespoon Worcestershire sauce
- 1 teaspoon dried thyme
- Salt and pepper to taste
- 2 tablespoons olive oil

Instructions:

1. In a large pot, heat olive oil over medium heat. Add beef stew meat and brown on all sides, about 5-7 minutes. Remove the beef from the pot and set it aside.

2. Add onion and garlic to the same pot and sauté for 2-3 minutes until they become fragrant.

3. Add beef broth, tomato paste, Worcestershire sauce, thyme, salt, and pepper to the pot. Stir well and bring it to a boil.

4. Add the browned beef, carrots, celery, and potatoes to the pot. Stir well, reduce heat to low and let it simmer for 2-3 hours or until the beef is tender.

5. Serve hot with crusty bread.

Nutritional Information:

This beef stew recipe makes 6 servings. Each serving contains approximately:

- 400 calories
- 35g protein
- 25g carbohydrates

- 18g fat
- 4g fiber

Tomato Soup

This creamy and flavorful **tomato soup** recipe is a classic that's always satisfying. It's made with ripe tomatoes, fresh herbs, and a touch of cream for a luxurious finish.

Ingredients:

- 2 lbs ripe tomatoes, chopped
- 1 onion, chopped
- 3 garlic cloves, minced
- 2 cups vegetable broth
- 1 cup heavy cream
- 2 tablespoons tomato paste
- 1 tablespoon dried basil
- 1 tablespoon dried oregano
- 1 tablespoon olive oil
- Salt and pepper to taste

Instructions:

1. In a large pot, heat olive oil over medium heat. Add onion and garlic and sauté for 2-3 minutes until they become fragrant.

2. Add chopped tomatoes, vegetable broth, tomato paste, basil, oregano, salt, and pepper to the pot. Stir well and bring it to a boil.

3. Reduce heat to low and let it simmer for 30-40 minutes or until the tomatoes are soft.

4. Remove the pot from heat and let it cool for a few minutes. Use an immersion blender to blend the

soup until smooth.

5. Add heavy cream to the pot and stir well. Heat the soup over low heat until it's warmed through.

6. Serve hot with croutons or a slice of bread.

Nutritional Information:

This tomato soup recipe makes 4 servings. Each serving contains approximately:

- 300 calories
- 6g protein
- 20g carbohydrates
- 25g fat
- 4g fiber

Salad recipes

Greek Salad

Description of the meal: Greek Salad is a healthy and refreshing dish that originates from Greece. It's a perfect combination of crunchy vegetables, salty feta cheese, and flavorful herbs. The dish is usually served as a side dish, but it can also be served as a main course.

Ingredients:

- 2 cups of cherry tomatoes, halved
- 1 cucumber, chopped
- 1 red onion, thinly sliced
- 1 green bell pepper, chopped

- 1/2 cup of Kalamata olives
- 1/2 cup of crumbled feta cheese
- 2 tablespoons of fresh parsley, chopped
- 1 tablespoon of fresh oregano, chopped
- 1/4 cup of olive oil
- 2 tablespoons of red wine vinegar
- Salt and pepper to taste

Instructions:

1. In a large bowl, combine the cherry tomatoes, cucumber, red onion, green bell pepper, and Kalamata olives.

2. In a small bowl, whisk together the olive oil, red wine vinegar, parsley, oregano, salt, and pepper.

3. Pour the dressing over the vegetables and toss to combine.

4. Sprinkle the crumbled feta cheese over the salad and serve immediately.

Nutritional Information:

- Calories: 220 kcal
- Total Fat: 18 g
- Saturated Fat: 5 g
- Cholesterol: 20 mg
- Total Carbohydrates: 11 g
- Dietary Fiber: 3 g
- Sugars: 5 g
- Protein: 5 g
- Sodium: 460 mg

Cobb Salad

Description of the meal: Cobb Salad is a classic American salad that is made with a variety of fresh ingredients. It's a hearty salad that can be served as a main course or as a side dish. The salad is usually made with chopped lettuce, tomatoes, bacon, avocado, and blue cheese, and is topped with a tangy dressing.

Ingredients:

- 6 cups of chopped romaine lettuce
- 2 cups of cooked chicken breast, chopped
- 2 medium tomatoes, chopped
- 2 hard-boiled eggs, chopped
- 1 avocado, chopped
- 4 strips of cooked bacon, chopped
- 1/2 cup of crumbled blue cheese
- 1/4 cup of red wine vinegar
- 2 tablespoons of Dijon mustard
- 1/2 cup of olive oil
- Salt and pepper to taste

Instructions:

1. In a large bowl, combine the chopped romaine lettuce, chopped chicken breast, chopped tomatoes, chopped hard-boiled eggs, chopped avocado, chopped bacon, and crumbled blue cheese.

2. In a small bowl, whisk together the red wine vinegar, Dijon mustard, olive oil, salt, and pepper.

3. Pour the dressing over the salad and toss to combine.

4. Serve immediately.

Nutritional Information:

- Calories: 560 kcal
- Total Fat: 47 g
- Saturated Fat: 10 g
- Cholesterol: 190 mg
- Total Carbohydrates: 10 g
- Dietary Fiber: 5 g
- Sugars: 2 g
- Protein: 28 g
- Sodium: 870 mg

Caprese Salad

Description of the meal: Caprese Salad is a simple and elegant Italian dish that is made with fresh mozzarella cheese, tomatoes, and basil. The salad is usually served as an appetizer or as a side dish.

Ingredients:

- 8 oz of fresh mozzarella cheese, sliced
- 2 medium tomatoes, sliced

Instructions:

1. On a large platter, arrange the sliced fresh mozzarella cheese and sliced tomatoes alternately.

2. Sprinkle fresh basil leaves over the cheese and tomato slices.

3. Drizzle olive oil over the salad.

4. Sprinkle salt and black pepper to taste.

5. Serve immediately.

Nutritional Information:

- Calories: 300 kcal
- Total Fat: 24 g
- Saturated Fat: 12 g
- Cholesterol: 70 mg
- Total Carbohydrates: 4 g
- Dietary Fiber: 1 g
- Sugars: 2 g
- Protein: 18 g
- Sodium: 570 mg

Waldorf Salad

Description of the meal: Waldorf Salad is a classic salad that originated in New York City. It's a sweet and savory salad that is made with apples, grapes, celery, and walnuts. The salad is usually served as a side dish.

Ingredients:

- 2 medium apples, chopped
- 1 cup of red grapes, halved
- 1/2 cup of celery, chopped
- 1/2 cup of walnuts, chopped
- 1/2 cup of mayonnaise
- 2 tablespoons of lemon juice
- 1 tablespoon of honey
- Salt and pepper to taste

Instructions:

1. In a large bowl, combine the chopped apples, halved red grapes, chopped celery, and chopped walnuts.

2. In a small bowl, whisk together the mayonnaise,

lemon juice, honey, salt, and pepper.

3. Pour the dressing over the salad and toss to combine.

4. Serve immediately.

Nutritional Information:

- Calories: 360 kcal
- Total Fat: 31 g
- Saturated Fat: 4 g
- Cholesterol: 10 mg
- Total Carbohydrates: 21 g
- Dietary Fiber: 3 g
- Sugars: 16 g
- Protein: 3 g
- Sodium: 170 mg

Sandwich and wrap recipes

BLT Sandwich

This classic sandwich combines crispy bacon, juicy tomato, and crisp lettuce on toasted bread slathered with mayo. Here's how to make it:

Ingredients:

- 2 slices of bread
- 3 strips of bacon
- 1/2 a tomato, sliced
- A handful of lettuce
- 1 tbsp mayonnaise

Instructions:

1. Cook the bacon in a skillet over medium heat until crispy.

2. Toast the bread to your liking.

3. Spread the mayonnaise on one or both slices of bread.

4. Layer the bacon, tomato, and lettuce on one slice of bread.

5. Top with the other slice of bread and slice in half.

Nutritional Information:

This BLT sandwich has approximately 420 calories, 25g fat, 30g carbohydrates, and 17g protein.

Veggie and Hummus Wrap

This delicious and healthy wrap is loaded with fresh veggies and creamy hummus for a satisfying lunch or dinner option. Here's how to make it:

Ingredients:

- 1 large tortilla wrap
- 1/4 cup hummus
- 1/4 cup shredded carrots
- 1/4 cup sliced cucumber
- 1/4 cup sliced bell pepper
- A handful of baby spinach

Instructions:

1. Spread the hummus on the tortilla wrap.

2. Layer the shredded carrots, sliced cucumber, sliced bell pepper, and baby spinach on top of the hummus.

3. Roll up the wrap tightly, tucking in the sides as you go.

4. Slice in half and serve.

Nutritional Information:

This veggie and hummus wrap has approximately 320 calories, 12g fat, 43g carbohydrates, and 11g protein.

Chicken Caesar Wrap

This flavorful wrap features tender chicken, crisp romaine lettuce, and a tangy Caesar dressing all wrapped up in a tortilla. Here's how to make it:

Ingredients:

- 1 large tortilla wrap
- 1 cooked chicken breast, sliced
- 1/2 cup romaine lettuce, chopped
- 1 tbsp Caesar dressing

Instructions:

1. Lay the tortilla wrap flat.

2. Spread the Caesar dressing on the tortilla wrap.

3. Layer the sliced chicken and chopped romaine lettuce on top of the dressing.

4. Roll up the wrap tightly, tucking in the sides as you go.

5. Slice in half and serve.

Nutritional Information:

This chicken Caesar wrap has approximately 350 calories, 14g fat, 29g carbohydrates, and 28g protein.

Grilled Cheese Sandwich

This classic sandwich is a comfort food favorite, with gooey melted cheese between two slices of buttery toasted bread. Here's how to make it:

Ingredients:

- 2 slices of bread
- 2 slices of cheese
- 1 tbsp butter

Instructions:

1. Heat a skillet over medium heat.
2. Butter one side of each slice of bread.
3. Place one slice of bread in the skillet, buttered side down.
4. Add the cheese slices on top of the bread.
5. Top with the other slice of bread, buttered side up.
6. Cook for 2-3 minutes per side, or until the bread is golden brown and the cheese is melted.
7. Slice in half and serve.

Nutritional Information:

This grilled cheese sandwich has approximately 450 calories, 25g fat, 35g carbohydrates, and 20g protein.

CHAPTER FOUR

Dinner Recipes

Dinner recipes that are easy to digest

Ginger Soy Glazed Salmon

This dish is a delicious and healthy meal that is perfect for a weeknight dinner or a special occasion. The salmon is marinated in a flavorful ginger soy glaze and then baked to perfection.

Ingredients:

- 4 salmon fillets
- 1/4 cup soy sauce
- 1/4 cup honey
- 1/4 cup rice vinegar
- 2 tbsp minced fresh ginger
- 2 cloves minced garlic
- 1/4 tsp red pepper flakes
- 1 tbsp vegetable oil
- Salt and pepper to taste
- Sliced green onions and sesame seeds for garnish

Instructions:

1. Preheat the oven to 400°F.
2. In a small bowl, whisk together the soy sauce, honey, rice vinegar, ginger, garlic, red pepper

flakes, vegetable oil, salt and pepper.

3. Place the salmon fillets in a baking dish and pour the marinade over them.

4. Bake for 12-15 minutes, or until the salmon is cooked through and flakes easily with a fork.

5. Garnish with sliced green onions and sesame seeds before serving.

Nutritional Information:

- Calories: 330
- Fat: 16g
- Protein: 34g
- Carbohydrates: 14g
- Fiber: 0g

Miso Soup with Tofu and Vegetables

This Japanese-inspired soup is warm, comforting, and packed with nutritious vegetables and tofu. The savory miso broth adds depth of flavor and richness to the dish.

Ingredients:

- 4 cups water
- 4 tbsp miso paste
- 1 tbsp vegetable oil
- 1 tbsp minced garlic
- 1 tbsp minced ginger
- 2 cups sliced mixed vegetables (such as mushrooms, bok choy, carrots, and snow peas)
- 1/2 block of firm tofu, cubed
- 2 green onions, thinly sliced
- Salt and pepper to taste

Instructions:

1. In a large pot, bring the water to a boil.

2. Reduce the heat to low and whisk in the miso paste until it dissolves completely.

3. In a separate skillet, heat the vegetable oil over medium-high heat. Add the garlic and ginger and sauté until fragrant, about 1-2 minutes.

4. Add the mixed vegetables and tofu to the skillet and sauté for another 5-7 minutes, or until the vegetables are tender and the tofu is lightly browned.

5. Add the vegetable and tofu mixture to the pot with the miso broth and stir to combine.

6. Season with salt and pepper to taste.

7. Garnish with sliced green onions before serving.

Nutritional Information:

- Calories: 170
- Fat: 8g
- Protein: 12g
- Carbohydrates: 14g
- Fiber: 4g

Lemon Garlic Shrimp and Broccoli

This zesty and flavorful dish is perfect for a quick and easy weeknight dinner. The shrimp and broccoli are cooked in a lemon garlic sauce that is both tangy and savory.

Ingredients:

- 1 lb raw shrimp, peeled and deveined
- 1 head of broccoli, cut into florets

- 2 tbsp olive oil
- 2 tbsp minced garlic
- 1/4 cup fresh lemon juice
- 1/4 cup chicken broth
- Salt and pepper to taste
- Chopped fresh parsley for garnish

Instructions:

1. In a large skillet, heat the olive oil over medium-high heat.

2. Add the minced garlic to the skillet and sauté until fragrant, about 1-2 minutes.

3. Add the broccoli florets to the skillet and sauté for another 5-7 minutes, or until the broccoli is tender-crisp.

4. Add the shrimp to the skillet and cook for another 2-3 minutes, or until they are pink and cooked through.

5. Pour in the lemon juice and chicken broth and stir to combine.

6. Season with salt and pepper to taste.

7. Garnish with chopped fresh parsley before serving.

Nutritional Information:

- Calories: 230
- Fat: 10g
- Protein: 28g
- Carbohydrates: 11g
- Fiber: 4g

Baked Chicken and Sweet Potatoes

This hearty and flavorful dish is perfect for a cozy dinner at home. The chicken and sweet potatoes are baked together in a savory spice mixture that is both delicious and aromatic.

Ingredients:

- 4 chicken breasts
- 2 large sweet potatoes, peeled and cubed
- 2 tbsp olive oil
- 2 tsp smoked paprika
- 1 tsp garlic powder
- 1 tsp onion powder
- 1 tsp dried thyme
- 1 tsp dried rosemary
- Salt and pepper to taste

Instructions:

1. Preheat the oven to 400°F.

2. In a small bowl, mix together the smoked paprika, garlic powder, onion powder, dried thyme, dried rosemary, salt, and pepper.

3. In a large baking dish, toss the cubed sweet potatoes with 1 tbsp of olive oil and half of the spice mixture.

4. Arrange the chicken breasts on top of the sweet potatoes and drizzle with the remaining 1 tbsp of olive oil.

5. Sprinkle the remaining spice mixture over the chicken breasts.

6. Bake for 30-35 minutes, or until the chicken is cooked through and the sweet potatoes are tender.

7. Serve hot.

Nutritional Information:

- Calories: 350
- Fat: 10g
- Protein: 35g
- Carbohydrates: 25g
- Fiber: 5g

One-pot meals

Turkey and Quinoa Stuffed Bell Peppers

This recipe for Turkey and Quinoa Stuffed Bell Peppers is a nutritious and flavorful meal that's perfect for a family dinner. The bell peppers are stuffed with a mixture of ground turkey, quinoa, vegetables, and spices, making them a tasty and healthy option.

Ingredients:

- 4 large bell peppers
- 1 pound ground turkey
- 1 cup quinoa, cooked
- 1 onion, chopped
- 2 garlic cloves, minced
- 1 tablespoon olive oil
- 1 teaspoon paprika
- 1 teaspoon cumin

- Salt and pepper, to taste
- 1 cup tomato sauce
- 1/2 cup shredded cheddar cheese

Instructions:

1. Preheat the oven to 375°F.

2. Cut off the tops of the bell peppers and remove the seeds and membranes.

3. In a large skillet, heat olive oil over medium heat. Add onion and garlic and cook for 2-3 minutes until softened.

4. Add ground turkey to the skillet and cook until browned.

5. Add cooked quinoa, paprika, cumin, salt, and pepper to the skillet and stir until well combined.

6. Pour tomato sauce into the skillet and stir to combine.

7. Stuff the bell peppers with the turkey and quinoa mixture.

8. Place the stuffed bell peppers in a baking dish and bake for 25 minutes.

9. Sprinkle shredded cheddar cheese on top of the bell peppers and bake for an additional 5 minutes until the cheese is melted and bubbly.

Nutritional Information:

- Calories: 390
- Fat: 17g
- Carbohydrates: 34g
- Protein: 28g

Creamy Tomato and Spinach Pasta

This Creamy Tomato and Spinach Pasta recipe is a quick and easy meal that's perfect for busy weeknights. The creamy tomato sauce is made with canned tomatoes, spinach, garlic, and cream, and it's a delicious way to add more vegetables to your diet.

Ingredients:

- 8 ounces pasta
- 1 tablespoon olive oil
- 2 garlic cloves, minced
- 1 can diced tomatoes
- 1/2 cup heavy cream
- 2 cups spinach leaves
- Salt and pepper, to taste
- Parmesan cheese, for serving

Instructions:

1. Cook pasta according to package instructions.

2. In a large skillet, heat olive oil over medium heat. Add garlic and cook for 1-2 minutes until fragrant.

3. Add canned tomatoes to the skillet and bring to a simmer.

4. Stir in heavy cream and spinach leaves and cook for 2-3 minutes until the spinach is wilted.

5. Season with salt and pepper to taste.

6. Drain pasta and add it to the skillet with the tomato sauce. Toss until well coated.

7. Serve with grated Parmesan cheese.

Nutritional Information:

- Calories: 475
- Fat: 23g
- Carbohydrates: 54g
- Protein: 14g

One-Pot Chicken and Rice

This One-Pot Chicken and Rice recipe is a comforting and satisfying meal that's perfect for a chilly evening. The dish is made in just one pot, which makes cleanup a breeze.

Ingredients:

- 1 pound boneless, skinless chicken breasts, cut into bite-sized pieces
- 1 tablespoon olive oil
- 1 onion, chopped
- 2 garlic cloves, minced
- 1 cup long-grain white rice
- 2 cups chicken broth
- 1 can diced tomatoes
- 1 teaspoon dried thyme
- Salt and pepper, to taste
- Fresh parsley, for garnish

Instructions:

1. In a large pot or Dutch oven, heat olive oil over medium heat. Add onion and garlic and cook for 2-3 minutes until softened.
2. Add chicken to the pot and cook until browned on all sides.

3. Add rice, chicken broth, canned tomatoes, thyme, salt, and pepper to the pot and stir until well combined.

4. Bring the mixture to a simmer and cover the pot with a lid.

5. Cook for 20-25 minutes, stirring occasionally, until the rice is tender and the liquid has been absorbed.

6. Remove from heat and let the mixture sit for 5 minutes before serving.

7. Garnish with fresh parsley.

Nutritional Information:

- Calories: 385
- Fat: 7g
- Carbohydrates: 49g
- Protein: 32g

Vegetable Quinoa Soup

This Vegetable Quinoa Soup is a healthy and delicious way to get more vegetables and protein in your diet. The soup is made with quinoa, a protein-packed grain, and a variety of vegetables, making it a filling and nutritious meal.

Ingredients:

- 1 tablespoon olive oil
- 1 onion, chopped
- 2 garlic cloves, minced
- 4 cups vegetable broth
- 1 can diced tomatoes
- 1 cup quinoa, rinsed

- 2 cups chopped mixed vegetables (carrots, celery, zucchini, etc.)
- 1 teaspoon dried thyme
- Salt and pepper, to taste
- Fresh parsley, for garnish

Instructions:

1. In a large pot or Dutch oven, heat olive oil over medium heat. Add onion and garlic and cook for 2-3 minutes until softened.

2. Add vegetable broth, canned tomatoes, quinoa, mixed vegetables, thyme, salt, and pepper to the pot and stir until well combined.

3. Bring the mixture to a simmer and cover the pot with a lid.

4. Cook for 20-25 minutes, stirring occasionally, until the quinoa and vegetables are tender.

5. Remove from heat and let the soup sit for 5 minutes before serving.

6. Garnish with fresh parsley.

Nutritional Information:

- Calories: 260
- Fat: 6g
- Carbohydrates: 42g
- Protein: 10g

Meat and fish dishes

Ginger Soy Glazed Salmon

This delicious and healthy meal is perfect for seafood

lovers. The Ginger Soy Glazed Salmon is a flavorful and savory dish that is easy to prepare. The salmon is marinated in a mixture of ginger, soy sauce, honey, and garlic to give it a rich and tangy taste. It is then baked to perfection and served with steamed vegetables for a complete meal.

Ingredients:

- 4 salmon fillets
- 1/4 cup low-sodium soy sauce
- 2 tbsp honey
- 2 tbsp grated ginger
- 2 garlic cloves, minced
- 1 tbsp olive oil
- Salt and pepper
- Steamed vegetables, for serving

Instructions:

1. Preheat the oven to 400°F.
2. In a small bowl, whisk together soy sauce, honey, ginger, garlic, and olive oil.
3. Season salmon fillets with salt and pepper.
4. Brush the marinade on top of the salmon.
5. Bake for 12-15 minutes, or until the salmon is cooked through.
6. Serve with steamed vegetables.

Nutritional Information:

- Calories: 350
- Fat: 18g
- Carbohydrates: 12g

- Protein: 35g

Lemon Garlic Shrimp and Broccoli

This meal is a quick and easy weeknight dinner that is packed with flavor. Lemon Garlic Shrimp and Broccoli is a healthy and satisfying dish that is ready in less than 30 minutes. The shrimp is marinated in a mixture of lemon juice, garlic, and olive oil, which gives it a zesty flavor. The broccoli is lightly steamed to retain its nutrients, and both are combined for a delicious and nutritious meal.

Ingredients:

- 1 lb shrimp, peeled and deveined
- 3 garlic cloves, minced
- 2 tbsp olive oil
- 2 tbsp lemon juice
- 1/2 tsp salt
- 1/4 tsp black pepper
- 1 lb broccoli florets

Instructions:

1. In a small bowl, whisk together garlic, olive oil, lemon juice, salt, and black pepper.

2. Add the shrimp to the bowl and toss to coat.

3. Heat a large skillet over medium-high heat.

4. Add the shrimp and cook until pink, about 2-3 minutes per side.

5. Remove the shrimp from the skillet and set aside.

6. Add the broccoli to the same skillet and cook until tender, about 5-7 minutes.

7. Add the shrimp back to the skillet and toss with

the broccoli.

8. Serve immediately.

Nutritional Information:

- Calories: 270
- Fat: 12g
- Carbohydrates: 11g
- Protein: 30g

Baked Chicken and Sweet Potatoes

Baked Chicken and Sweet Potatoes is a hearty and healthy meal that is perfect for any night of the week. The chicken is seasoned with a blend of herbs and spices and baked until golden brown. The sweet potatoes are roasted to perfection, giving them a slightly caramelized flavor. This dish is high in protein and loaded with vitamins and minerals, making it a great choice for a healthy dinner.

Ingredients:

- 4 bone-in, skin-on chicken thighs
- 2 sweet potatoes, peeled and chopped
- 2 tbsp olive oil
- 1 tbsp garlic powder
- 1 tbsp dried thyme
- 1 tbsp paprika
- Salt and pepper

Instructions:

1. Preheat the oven to 425°F.
2. In a small bowl, mix together garlic powder, dried

thyme, paprika, salt, and pepper.

3. Rub the chicken thighs with the seasoning mixture, making sure to coat them well.
4. In a large baking dish, arrange the chicken thighs and sweet potato chunks in a single layer.
5. Drizzle olive oil over the chicken and sweet potatoes.
6. Bake for 35-40 minutes, or until the chicken is cooked through and the sweet potatoes are tender and lightly caramelized.
7. Serve hot.

Nutritional Information:

- Calories: 380
- Fat: 21g
- Carbohydrates: 21g
- Protein: 27g

Beef and Broccoli Stir-Fry

This Beef and Broccoli Stir-Fry is a quick and easy meal that is perfect for busy weeknights. The beef is marinated in a mixture of soy sauce, garlic, and ginger, and then stir-fried with broccoli and other vegetables for a flavorful and healthy dish. Serve it over rice or noodles for a complete meal.

Ingredients:

- 1 lb flank steak, thinly sliced
- 1/4 cup low-sodium soy sauce
- 2 garlic cloves, minced
- 1 tbsp grated ginger
- 1 tbsp cornstarch
- 2 tbsp vegetable oil

- 1 broccoli head, chopped into florets
- 1 red bell pepper, sliced
- 1 onion, sliced
- Salt and pepper

Instructions:

1. In a small bowl, whisk together soy sauce, garlic, ginger, and cornstarch.
2. Add the beef to the bowl and toss to coat.
3. Heat 1 tablespoon of vegetable oil in a large skillet or wok over high heat.
4. Add the beef to the skillet and stir-fry until browned, about 3-4 minutes.
5. Remove the beef from the skillet and set aside.
6. Heat the remaining tablespoon of oil in the skillet.
7. Add the broccoli, red bell pepper, and onion to the skillet and stir-fry until the vegetables are tender, about 5-7 minutes.
8. Add the beef back to the skillet and toss with the vegetables.
9. Season with salt and pepper, to taste.
10. Serve over rice or noodles.

Nutritional Information:

- Calories: 390
- Fat: 19g
- Carbohydrates: 20g
- Protein: 36g

Vegetable dishes

Roasted Vegetable Lasagna

This vegetarian lasagna is a great way to incorporate vegetables into your meal. Roasted vegetables, including zucchini, eggplant, and bell peppers, are layered between lasagna noodles and a creamy ricotta cheese mixture.

Ingredients:

- 1 large zucchini, sliced
- 1 large eggplant, sliced
- 1 red bell pepper, sliced
- 1 yellow bell pepper, sliced
- 1 package lasagna noodles
- 1 container ricotta cheese
- 1 egg
- 1/2 cup grated Parmesan cheese
- 2 cups shredded mozzarella cheese
- 1 jar pasta sauce

Instructions:

1. Preheat oven to 400°F (200°C).

2. Place sliced vegetables on a baking sheet, drizzle with olive oil, and sprinkle with salt and pepper. Roast in the oven for 20-25 minutes, until tender.

3. Cook lasagna noodles according to package directions.

4. In a bowl, mix together ricotta cheese, egg, and

Parmesan cheese.

5. Spread a layer of pasta sauce on the bottom of a 9x13 inch baking dish. Layer lasagna noodles on top, followed by a layer of roasted vegetables, a layer of ricotta cheese mixture, and a layer of shredded mozzarella cheese. Repeat until all ingredients are used up.

6. Cover the baking dish with foil and bake in the oven for 30 minutes. Remove foil and bake for an additional 10-15 minutes, until cheese is melted and bubbly.

7. Let lasagna cool for a few minutes before serving.

Nutritional Information:

- Calories: 400
- Fat: 16g
- Carbohydrates: 42g
- Protein: 22g

Miso Soup with Tofu and Vegetables

Miso soup is a traditional Japanese soup made with a miso paste broth and ingredients such as tofu and seaweed. This version is packed with vegetables and makes for a healthy and satisfying meal.

Ingredients:

- 4 cups vegetable broth
- 2 tablespoons miso paste
- 1 tablespoon soy sauce
- 1 tablespoon rice vinegar
- 1 teaspoon grated ginger
- 1 cup sliced mushrooms

- 1 cup chopped bok choy
- 1/2 cup sliced scallions
- 1/2 cup diced firm tofu
- 1 sheet nori seaweed, cut into small pieces

Instructions:

1. In a pot, bring vegetable broth to a simmer.

2. In a small bowl, whisk together miso paste, soy sauce, rice vinegar, and grated ginger. Add to the pot and stir to combine.

3. Add sliced mushrooms, chopped bok choy, sliced scallions, diced tofu, and cut-up nori seaweed to the pot. Simmer for 5-7 minutes, until vegetables are tender and tofu is heated through.

4. Serve hot.

Nutritional Information:

- Calories: 150
- Fat: 5g
- Carbohydrates: 17g
- Protein: 11g

Creamy Tomato and Spinach Pasta

This creamy pasta dish is a comforting and delicious meal that is perfect for a weeknight dinner. The combination of tomato sauce and spinach gives this dish a healthy twist.

Ingredients:

- 1 pound penne pasta
- 1 tablespoon olive oil

- 1 onion, chopped
- 2 cloves garlic, minced
- 1 can (28 ounces) crushed tomatoes
- 1/2 cup heavy cream
- 1/2 cup grated Parmesan cheese
- 2 cups fresh spinach
- Salt and pepper to taste

Instructions:

1. Cook pasta according to package directions. Drain and set aside.

2. In a large skillet, heat olive oil over medium heat. Add chopped onion and minced garlic and cook until softened, about 5 minutes.

3. Add crushed tomatoes to the skillet and bring to a simmer. Let cook for 10-15 minutes, until sauce has thickened.

4. Stir in heavy cream and grated Parmesan cheese. Add fresh spinach and stir until spinach has wilted.

5. Add cooked pasta to the skillet and toss with sauce until pasta is coated evenly. Season with salt and pepper to taste.

6. Serve hot.

Nutritional Information:

- Calories: 500
- Fat: 18g
- Carbohydrates: 68g
- Protein: 18g

Vegetable Quinoa Soup

This healthy and hearty vegetable quinoa soup is packed with nutrients and makes for a filling meal. It is perfect for a cold day or when you need something comforting and satisfying.

Ingredients:

- 1 tablespoon olive oil
- 1 onion, chopped
- 2 cloves garlic, minced
- 2 carrots, diced
- 2 stalks celery, diced
- 1 can (14 ounces) diced tomatoes
- 1 can (15 ounces) chickpeas, drained and rinsed
- 1 cup quinoa, rinsed
- 6 cups vegetable broth
- 1 teaspoon dried thyme
- 1/2 teaspoon paprika
- Salt and pepper to taste

Instructions:

1. In a large pot, heat olive oil over medium heat. Add chopped onion and minced garlic and cook until softened, about 5 minutes.

2. Add diced carrots and celery to the pot and cook until vegetables are tender, about 10 minutes.

3. Add diced tomatoes, chickpeas, quinoa, vegetable broth, dried thyme, and paprika to the pot. Bring to a simmer and let cook for 20-25 minutes, until quinoa is cooked through.

4. Season with salt and pepper to taste.

5. Serve hot.

Nutritional Information:

- Calories: 350
- Fat: 7g
- Carbohydrates: 56g
- Protein: 14g

CHAPTER FIVE

Snack Recipes

Snacks that are easy to digest

Rice cakes with almond butter and sliced banana

This meal is a delicious and healthy snack option that is perfect for anyone looking for a quick and easy bite to eat. Rice cakes are low in calories and are a great source of fiber and complex carbohydrates. Almond butter is a healthy fat that is high in protein, while bananas are a great source of potassium and vitamin C.

Ingredients:

- 2 rice cakes
- 2 tablespoons almond butter
- 1 banana, sliced

Instructions:

1. Spread 1 tablespoon of almond butter on each rice cake.
2. Top each rice cake with sliced banana.
3. Serve and enjoy!

Nutritional Information:

- Calories: 300
- Fat: 10g
- Carbohydrates: 48g

- Fiber: 6g
- Protein: 6g

Roasted sweet potato wedges with Greek yogurt dip

This meal is a healthy and satisfying option that is perfect for a quick lunch or snack. Sweet potatoes are a great source of fiber and vitamins, while Greek yogurt is high in protein and low in calories.

Ingredients:

- 1 large sweet potato, cut into wedges
- 1 tablespoon olive oil
- 1/2 teaspoon paprika
- 1/4 teaspoon garlic powder
- Salt and pepper to taste
- 1/2 cup Greek yogurt
- 1/2 teaspoon lemon juice
- 1/4 teaspoon dried dill

Instructions:

1. Preheat oven to 400°F (200°C).

2. Toss sweet potato wedges in olive oil, paprika, garlic powder, salt, and pepper.

3. Place sweet potato wedges on a baking sheet and bake for 20-25 minutes, or until tender and golden brown.

4. While the sweet potatoes are roasting, mix together Greek yogurt, lemon juice, and dried dill in a small bowl.

5. Serve sweet potato wedges with Greek yogurt dip on the side.

Nutritional Information:

- Calories: 200
- Fat: 6g
- Carbohydrates: 32g
- Fiber: 6g
- Protein: 8g

Boiled or steamed edamame with a sprinkle of sea salt

This meal is a simple and nutritious snack that is packed with protein and fiber. Edamame is a type of soybean that is often served as an appetizer in Japanese cuisine.

Ingredients:

- 1 cup edamame
- 1/4 teaspoon sea salt

Instructions:

1. Bring a pot of salted water to a boil.
2. Add edamame to the boiling water and cook for 5-7 minutes, or until tender.
3. Drain edamame and sprinkle with sea salt.
4. Serve and enjoy!

Nutritional Information:

- Calories: 120
- Fat: 5g
- Carbohydrates: 8g
- Fiber: 4g
- Protein: 12g

Toasted sourdough with avocado mash and cherry tomatoes

This meal is a delicious and filling option that is perfect for breakfast, lunch, or a snack. Sourdough bread is a great source of complex carbohydrates, while avocado is high in healthy fats and fiber. Cherry tomatoes are a great source of vitamin C and add a pop of color to this dish.

Ingredients:

- 2 slices sourdough bread
- 1 avocado, mashed
- 1/2 cup cherry tomatoes, halved
- Salt and pepper to taste

Instructions:

1. Toast sourdough bread until golden brown.
2. Mash avocado in a small bowl and season with salt and pepper to taste.
3. Spread the avocado mash on each slice of toasted sourdough. 4. Top the avocado mash with halved cherry tomatoes.
5. Serve and enjoy!

Nutritional Information:

- Calories: 400
- Fat: 18g
- Carbohydrates: 50g
- Fiber: 10g
- Protein: 12g

Fruit and vegetable snacks

Apple slices with almond butter and cinnamon

This snack is a perfect balance of sweet and nutty flavors that will keep you satisfied and energized throughout the day.

Ingredients

- 1 medium-sized apple
- 1 tablespoon almond butter
- 1/2 teaspoon cinnamon

Instructions

1. Wash and core the apple, then slice it into thin pieces.
2. Spread the almond butter on each slice of apple.
3. Sprinkle cinnamon on top of the almond butter.
4. Serve and enjoy!

Nutritional Information

- Calories: 163
- Fat: 8g
- Carbohydrates: 24g
- Protein: 2g

Carrot sticks with hummus dip

This snack is a great source of fiber, protein, and healthy fats that will keep you feeling full and satisfied for longer periods of time.

Ingredients

- 2 medium-sized carrots
- 2 tablespoons hummus

Instructions

1. Peel the carrots and cut them into sticks.
2. Serve the carrot sticks with hummus on the side for dipping.

Nutritional Information

- Calories: 84
- Fat: 4g
- Carbohydrates: 12g
- Protein: 3g

Frozen grapes

This snack is a refreshing and simple way to cool down on a hot day.

Ingredients

- 1 cup seedless grapes

Instructions

1. Wash the grapes and remove any stems.
2. Place the grapes in a freezer-safe container and freeze for at least 2 hours.
3. Serve and enjoy!

Nutritional Information

- Calories: 62
- Fat: 0g
- Carbohydrates: 16g
- Protein: 1g

Cucumber slices with tzatziki dip

This snack is a light and refreshing way to get your daily dose of vegetables and protein.

Ingredients

- 1 medium-sized cucumber
- 1/4 cup tzatziki dip

Instructions

1. Wash the cucumber and slice it into thin pieces.
2. Serve the cucumber slices with tzatziki dip on the side for dipping.

Nutritional Information

- Calories: 41
- Fat: 2g
- Carbohydrates: 4g
- Protein: 2g

Nut and seed snacks

Trail Mix with Almonds, Pumpkin Seeds, and Dried Cranberries

This trail mix is a perfect snack for those who are always on the go. It's a combination of crunchy almonds, nutritious pumpkin seeds, and sweet dried cranberries.

Ingredients:

- 1 cup almonds
- 1/2 cup pumpkin seeds
- 1/2 cup dried cranberries

Instructions:

1. Preheat your oven to 350°F (175°C).
2. Spread the almonds and pumpkin seeds on a baking sheet and bake for 8-10 minutes or until lightly golden and fragrant.
3. Let the almonds and pumpkin seeds cool completely.
4. Once cooled, mix the almonds, pumpkin seeds, and dried cranberries together.

5. Store the trail mix in an airtight container.

Nutritional Information:

- Calories: 200
- Protein: 6g
- Fat: 15g
- Carbohydrates: 13g
- Fiber: 4g

Peanut Butter and Jelly Energy Balls

These energy balls are a delicious and nutritious snack that is perfect for an afternoon pick-me-up. They are made with natural peanut butter, oats, and jam.

Ingredients:

- 1 cup rolled oats
- 1/2 cup natural peanut butter
- 1/4 cup jam (your favorite flavor)

Instructions:

1. In a large bowl, mix together the oats, peanut butter, and jam until well combined.

2. Form the mixture into balls (about 1 tablespoon each).

3. Place the energy balls on a baking sheet lined with parchment paper.

4. Refrigerate the energy balls for at least 30 minutes or until firm.

5. Store the energy balls in an airtight container in the refrigerator.

Nutritional Information:

- Calories: 150

- Protein: 5g
- Fat: 7g
- Carbohydrates: 18g
- Fiber: 2g

Cashew and Coconut Date Bites

These cashew and coconut date bites are a delicious and healthy snack that is perfect for satisfying your sweet tooth. They are made with simple ingredients and are naturally sweetened with dates.

Ingredients:

- 1 cup raw cashews
- 1 cup unsweetened shredded coconut
- 10 Medjool dates, pitted
- 1/4 tsp salt

Instructions:

1. In a food processor, pulse the cashews and shredded coconut until finely ground.

2. Add the pitted dates and salt to the food processor and pulse until the mixture forms a sticky dough.

3. Form the mixture into small balls (about 1 tablespoon each).

4. Store the cashew and coconut date bites in an airtight container in the refrigerator.

Nutritional Information:

- Calories: 120
- Protein: 2g
- Fat: 7g
- Carbohydrates: 14g

- Fiber: 2g

Sunflower Seed Butter and Honey Toast

This sunflower seed butter and honey toast is a simple and delicious breakfast or snack that is perfect for those who are looking for a quick and easy meal.

Ingredients:

- 2 slices whole-grain bread
- 2 tbsp sunflower seed butter
- 1 tbsp honey

Instructions:

1. Toast the slices of bread in a toaster.
2. Spread the sunflower seed butter evenly over each slice of toast.
3. Drizzle the honey over the sunflower seed butter.
4. Serve the sunflower seed butter and honey toast immediately.

Nutritional Information:

- Fat: 11g
- Carbohydrates: 43g
- Fiber: 6g
- Sugar: 15g
- Protein: 10g

Smoothie and drink recipes

Strawberry Banana Smoothie with Almond Milk

This refreshing **Strawberry Banana Smoothie with Almond Milk** is a healthy and delicious way to start your day. Packed with vitamins and minerals, this smoothie is easy to make and perfect for those on-the-go.

Ingredients:

- 1 cup fresh strawberries, hulled and sliced
- 1 medium banana, peeled and sliced
- 1 cup unsweetened almond milk
- 1/2 cup ice cubes

Instructions:

1. Add the strawberries, banana, almond milk, and ice cubes to a blender.
2. Blend until smooth and creamy.
3. Pour the smoothie into a glass and serve immediately.

Nutritional Information:

- Calories: 160
- Total Fat: 3g
- Saturated Fat: 0g
- Cholesterol: 0mg
- Sodium: 100mg
- Total Carbohydrates: 34g
- Dietary Fiber: 6g
- Sugars: 20g
- Protein: 3g

Pineapple Coconut Water Smoothie

This tropical **Pineapple Coconut Water Smoothie** is a great way to hydrate and energize your body. It is a healthy and refreshing drink that is perfect for those hot summer days.

Ingredients:

- 2 cups fresh pineapple chunks
- 1 cup coconut water
- 1 banana, peeled and sliced
- 1/2 cup ice cubes

Instructions:

1. Add the pineapple chunks, coconut water, banana, and ice cubes to a blender.

2. Blend until smooth and creamy.

3. Pour the smoothie into a glass and serve immediately.

Nutritional Information:

- Calories: 170
- Total Fat: 1.5g
- Saturated Fat: 1g
- Cholesterol: 0mg
- Sodium: 60mg
- Total Carbohydrates: 40g
- Dietary Fiber: 5g
- Sugars: 26g
- Protein: 2g

Chocolate Peanut Butter Protein Shake

This **Chocolate Peanut Butter Protein Shake** is a delicious and nutritious way to satisfy your sweet tooth and fuel your body with protein. It is perfect for post-workout recovery or as a quick breakfast on-the-go.

Ingredients:

- 1 scoop chocolate protein powder

- 1 tablespoon peanut butter
- 1 medium banana, peeled and sliced
- 1 cup unsweetened almond milk
- 1/2 cup ice cubes

Instructions:

1. Add the chocolate protein powder, peanut butter, banana, almond milk, and ice cubes to a blender.

2. Blend until smooth and creamy.

3. Pour the protein shake into a glass and serve immediately.

Nutritional Information:

- Calories: 320
- Total Fat: 12g
- Saturated Fat: 2g
- Cholesterol: 25mg
- Sodium: 340mg
- Total Carbohydrates: 27g
- Dietary Fiber: 6g
- Sugars: 14g
- Protein: 31g

Matcha Green Tea Latte with Almond Milk

This **Matcha Green Tea Latte with Almond Milk** is a healthy and delicious way to enjoy the benefits of matcha. Matcha is a type of green tea that is packed with antioxidants and provides a natural energy boost.

Ingredients:

- 1 teaspoon matcha powder
- 1 cup unsweetened almond milk

- 1 tablespoon honey or agave nectar (optional)
- 1/4 teaspoon vanilla extract (optional)

Instructions:

1. Heat the almond milk in a small saucepan over medium heat until it begins to steam. Do not boil.

2. In a small bowl, whisk together the matcha powder and 2 tablespoons of hot water until smooth.

3. Pour the matcha mixture into a mug.

4. Add the hot almond milk to the mug and stir to combine.

5. If desired, add honey or agave nectar and vanilla extract to taste.

6. Use a frother or whisk to create foam on top of the latte.

7. Serve immediately.

Nutritional Information:

- Calories: 60
- Total Fat: 2.5g
- Saturated Fat: 0g
- Cholesterol: 0mg
- Sodium: 170mg
- Total Carbohydrates: 9g
- Dietary Fiber: 1g
- Sugars: 6g
- Protein: 2g

CHAPTER SIX

Dessert Recipes

Low-fat and low-sugar dessert recipes

Low-Fat Lemon Sorbet

This Low-Fat Lemon Sorbet is a refreshing and healthy dessert that is perfect for hot summer days. Made with only a few simple ingredients, this sorbet is easy to prepare and can be enjoyed by everyone.

Ingredients:

- 2 cups water
- 1 cup freshly squeezed lemon juice
- 1/2 cup sugar
- 1 tablespoon lemon zest

Instructions:

1. In a saucepan, combine the water, sugar, and lemon zest. Bring to a boil over medium-high heat, stirring constantly, until the sugar is dissolved.

2. Reduce the heat and simmer for 5 minutes.

3. Remove from heat and let cool to room temperature.

4. Stir in the lemon juice.

5. Pour the mixture into a container and freeze for

2-3 hours, stirring occasionally, until the sorbet is set.

Nutritional Information:

- Serving size: 1/2 cup
- Calories: 75
- Fat: 0g
- Carbohydrates: 19g
- Fiber: 0g
- Protein: 0g

Baked Apples with Cinnamon and Honey

These Baked Apples with Cinnamon and Honey are a delicious and healthy dessert that is perfect for fall. The apples are tender and sweet, and the cinnamon and honey add a warm and comforting flavor.

Ingredients:

- 4 medium apples, cored
- 2 tablespoons honey
- 1 teaspoon ground cinnamon

Instructions:

1. Preheat the oven to 375°F (190°C).
2. Place the cored apples in a baking dish.
3. Drizzle honey over the apples.
4. Sprinkle cinnamon over the apples.
5. Bake for 25-30 minutes, or until the apples are tender and golden brown.
6. Serve warm.

Nutritional Information:

- Serving size: 1 apple
- Calories: 120
- Fat: 0g
- Carbohydrates: 32g
- Fiber: 5g
- Protein: 1g

Chocolate Chia Seed Pudding

This Chocolate Chia Seed Pudding is a healthy and satisfying dessert that is perfect for chocolate lovers. Made with chia seeds, almond milk, and cocoa powder, this pudding is rich and creamy, without any added sugar.

Ingredients:

- 1/4 cup chia seeds
- 1 cup unsweetened almond milk
- 2 tablespoons unsweetened cocoa powder
- 1/2 teaspoon vanilla extract
- 1-2 tablespoons honey (optional)

Instructions:

1. In a bowl, whisk together the chia seeds, almond milk, cocoa powder, and vanilla extract.
2. Cover and refrigerate for at least 2 hours, or overnight, until the mixture thickens.
3. Stir in the honey, if desired.
4. Serve chilled.

Nutritional Information:

- Serving size: 1/2 cup
- Calories: 120
- Fat: 7g

- Carbohydrates: 14g
- Fiber: 8g
- Protein: 5g

Puddings and custards

Vanilla Bean Custard

Description

This Vanilla Bean Custard is a classic dessert that is smooth, creamy and rich in flavor. Made with eggs, milk, sugar, and a vanilla bean, this dessert is perfect for any occasion.

Ingredients

- 1 cup milk
- 1 cup heavy cream
- 1 vanilla bean
- 3 egg yolks
- 1/4 cup sugar
- 1/4 tsp salt

Instructions

1. Preheat the oven to 300°F.

2. In a saucepan, heat the milk, cream, and vanilla bean until just simmering. Turn off the heat and let the mixture steep for 10 minutes.

3. In a separate bowl, whisk together the egg yolks, sugar, and salt until pale yellow.

4. Remove the vanilla bean from the milk mixture and scrape the seeds into the egg mixture. Whisk

to combine.

5. Slowly pour the hot milk mixture into the egg mixture, whisking constantly.

6. Strain the mixture through a fine-mesh sieve and pour it into 4 ramekins.

7. Place the ramekins in a baking dish and fill the dish with enough hot water to come halfway up the sides of the ramekins.

8. Bake for 30-35 minutes, or until the custard is set but still jiggles slightly in the center.

9. Remove from the oven and let cool to room temperature before serving.

Nutritional Information

- Calories: 250
- Fat: 18g
- Carbohydrates: 17g
- Protein: 5g

Rice Pudding with Raisins

Description

This Rice Pudding with Raisins is a comforting and delicious dessert that is perfect for a cozy night in. Made with simple ingredients like rice, milk, sugar, and raisins, this dessert is sure to satisfy your sweet tooth.

Ingredients

- 1 cup cooked rice
- 2 cups milk
- 1/2 cup sugar

- 1/2 cup raisins
- 1/2 tsp vanilla extract
- 1/4 tsp ground cinnamon
- Pinch of salt

Instructions

1. In a saucepan, combine the cooked rice, milk, sugar, raisins, vanilla extract, cinnamon, and salt.

2. Cook over medium heat, stirring occasionally, until the mixture comes to a simmer.

3. Reduce the heat to low and continue to cook, stirring occasionally, for 20-25 minutes or until the pudding has thickened.

4. Remove from the heat and let cool for 10 minutes before serving.

Nutritional Information

- Calories: 240
- Fat: 2g
- Carbohydrates: 52g
- Protein: 5g

Tapioca Pudding with Coconut Milk

Description

This Tapioca Pudding with Coconut Milk is a creamy and indulgent dessert that is perfect for anyone who loves tapioca. Made with tapioca pearls, coconut milk, and sugar, this dessert is sure to satisfy your sweet tooth.

Ingredients

- 1 cup tapioca pearls

- 4 cups water
- 1 can (13.5 oz) coconut milk
- 1/2 cup sugar
- Pinch of salt

Instructions

1. In a large pot, bring the water to a boil.
2. Add the tapioca pearls and cook for 10-12 minutes or until the pearls are translucent and tender.
3. Drain the tapioca pearls and rinse with cold water.
4. In a saucepan, combine the cooked tapioca pearls, coconutmilk, sugar, and salt.
5. Cook over medium heat, stirring constantly, until the mixture comes to a simmer.
6. Reduce the heat to low and continue to cook, stirring occasionally, for 15-20 minutes or until the pudding has thickened.
7. Remove from the heat and let cool for 10 minutes before serving.

Nutritional Information

- Calories: 340
- Fat: 16g
- Carbohydrates: 47g
- Protein: 3g

Fruit desserts

Vanilla Bean Custard

Description of the Meal: Vanilla bean custard is a delicious and creamy dessert that is perfect for any occasion. It has a smooth and silky texture that melts in your mouth and a rich vanilla flavor that is hard to resist.

Ingredients:

- 2 cups of heavy cream
- 1 vanilla bean
- 1/2 cup of sugar
- 6 egg yolks

Instructions:

1. Preheat the oven to 325°F (165°C).

2. In a medium saucepan, combine the heavy cream and vanilla bean (split and scraped). Heat the mixture over medium heat until it comes to a simmer.

3. In a mixing bowl, whisk together the sugar and egg yolks until pale and thick.

4. Slowly pour the hot cream into the egg mixture, whisking constantly to combine.

5. Strain the mixture through a fine-mesh sieve to remove any solids and divide it into six 4-ounce ramekins.

6. Place the ramekins in a baking dish and fill the dish with hot water until it reaches halfway up the sides of the ramekins.

7. Bake for 35-40 minutes, or until the custards are set but still slightly jiggly in the center.

8. Remove the ramekins from the water bath and let them cool to room temperature. Then, cover with plastic wrap and refrigerate for at least 2 hours.

9. Serve chilled and enjoy!

Nutritional Information:

- Calories: 460
- Fat: 39g
- Carbohydrates: 24g
- Protein: 5g

Rice Pudding with Raisins

Description of the Meal: Rice pudding with raisins is a classic and comforting dessert that is perfect for chilly nights. It has a creamy texture and a hint of cinnamon that makes it irresistible.

Ingredients:

- 1 cup of white rice
- 2 cups of water
- 1/2 teaspoon of salt
- 4 cups of milk
- 1/2 cup of sugar
- 1/2 cup of raisins
- 1 teaspoon of vanilla extract
- 1/2 teaspoon of ground cinnamon

Instructions:

1. In a medium saucepan, combine the rice, water, and salt. Bring to a boil over high heat, then reduce the heat to low, cover, and simmer for 18-20 minutes, or until the rice is cooked and the water is absorbed.

2. Add the milk, sugar, raisins, vanilla extract, and ground cinnamon to the saucepan with the rice.

Stir well to combine.

3. Increase the heat to medium and bring the mixture to a boil, stirring constantly to prevent the rice from sticking to the bottom of the pan.

4. Reduce the heat to low and let the rice pudding simmer for 25-30 minutes, or until the mixture thickens and the rice is soft and creamy.

5. Remove from heat and let it cool for a few minutes before serving.

6. Serve warm or chilled, and enjoy!

Nutritional Information:

- Calories: 370
- Fat: 6g
- Carbohydrates: 70g
- Protein: 11g

Tapioca Pudding with Coconut Milk

Description of the Meal: Tapioca pudding with coconut milk is a creamy and tropical dessert that is perfect for hot summer days. It has a unique texture and a delicate coconut flavor that will transport you to a tropical paradise.

Ingredients:

- 1/2 cup of small tapioca pearls
- 1 can (13.5 oz) of coconut milk
- 1/4 cup of sugar
- 1/4 teaspoon of salt
- 1/2 teaspoon of vanilla extract

- Fresh fruit or toasted coconut flakes for topping (optional)

Instructions:

1. Soak the tapioca pearls in cold water for at least 30 minutes, or until they are soft and translucent.

2. In a medium saucepan, combine the soaked tapioca pearls, coconut milk, sugar, and salt. Heat the mixture over medium heat, stirring constantly, until it comes to a boil.

3. Reduce the heat to low and let the pudding simmer for 10-15 minutes, or until the tapioca pearls are fully cooked and the pudding has thickened.

4. Remove the saucepan from the heat and stir in the vanilla extract.

5. Let the tapioca pudding cool to room temperature, then transfer it to a serving dish or individual bowls.

6. Chill in the refrigerator for at least 1 hour, or until fully set.

7. Top with fresh fruit or toasted coconut flakes, if desired, and enjoy!

Nutritional Information:

- Calories: 290
- Fat: 20g
- Carbohydrates: 25g
- Protein: 2g

Baked goods

Whole Wheat Banana Bread

This whole wheat banana bread is a delicious and healthy option for breakfast or a snack. Made with whole wheat flour and ripe bananas, it is a good source of fiber and potassium.

Ingredients

- 2 cups whole wheat flour
- 1 teaspoon baking soda
- 1/4 teaspoon salt
- 1/2 cup unsalted butter, softened
- 1/2 cup brown sugar
- 2 large eggs
- 3 ripe bananas, mashed
- 1 teaspoon vanilla extract

Instructions

1. Preheat the oven to 350°F (175°C). Grease a 9x5 inch loaf pan.

2. In a medium bowl, mix the whole wheat flour, baking soda, and salt together.

3. In a separate large bowl, cream together the butter and brown sugar until light and fluffy.

4. Beat in the eggs, one at a time, until well blended.

5. Add the mashed bananas and vanilla extract to the wet mixture and mix until combined.

6. Gradually stir in the dry mixture until just combined. Do not overmix.

7. Pour the batter into the prepared loaf pan and bake for 50-60 minutes, or until a toothpick

inserted into the center of the bread comes out clean.

8. Allow the bread to cool in the pan for 10 minutes before removing it and placing it on a wire rack to cool completely.

Nutritional Information

- Calories: 225
- Fat: 10g
- Carbohydrates: 33g
- Fiber: 4g
- Protein: 4g

Low-Fat Blueberry Muffins

These low-fat blueberry muffins are a healthier version of the classic breakfast treat. Made with low-fat yogurt and fresh blueberries, they are a good source of protein and antioxidants.

Ingredients

- 2 cups all-purpose flour
- 2 teaspoons baking powder
- 1/2 teaspoon salt
- 1/2 cup sugar
- 1/4 cup unsalted butter, melted and cooled
- 2 large eggs
- 1/2 cup low-fat plain yogurt
- 1/2 cup skim milk
- 1 teaspoon vanilla extract
- 1 cup fresh blueberries

Instructions

1. Preheat the oven to 375°F (190°C). Line a muffin tin with paper liners.
2. In a medium bowl, whisk together the flour, baking powder, and salt.
3. In a separate large bowl, whisk together the sugar and melted butter until well combined.
4. Add the eggs, one at a time, whisking well after each addition.
5. Whisk in the yogurt, milk, and vanilla extract until the mixture is smooth.
6. Gradually stir in the dry ingredients until just combined.
7. Gently fold in the blueberries.
8. Fill each muffin cup about 3/4 full with batter.
9. Bake for 18-20 minutes, or until a toothpick inserted into the center of a muffin comes out clean.
10. Allow the muffins to cool in the tin for 5 minutes before transferring them to a wire rack to cool completely.

Nutritional Information

- Calories: 150
- Fat: 3g
- Carbohydrates: 27g
- Fiber: 1g
- Protein: 4g

Apple Oatmeal Cookies

These apple oatmeal cookies are a nutritious and tasty

snack that can be enjoyed anytime of the day. Made with oats, whole wheat flour, and fresh apples, they are a good source of fiber and vitamins.

Ingredients

- 1 1/2 cups rolled oats
- 1 cup whole wheat flour
- 1/2 teaspoon baking soda
- 1/2 teaspoon ground cinnamon
- 1/4 teaspoon salt
- 1/2 cup unsalted butter, softened
- 1/2 cup brown sugar
- 1 large egg
- 1 teaspoon vanilla extract
- 1 cup grated apple (about 1 medium apple)
- 1/2 cup raisins

Instructions

1. Preheat the oven to 350°F (175°C). Line a baking sheet with parchment paper.

2. In a medium bowl, mix together the rolled oats, whole wheat flour, baking soda, cinnamon, and salt.

3. In a separate large bowl, cream together the butter and brown sugar until light and fluffy.

4. Beat in the egg and vanilla extract until well blended.

5. Gradually stir in the dry mixture until just combined.

6. Fold in the grated apple and raisins until evenly

distributed.

7. Drop spoonfuls of the dough onto the prepared baking sheet, leaving about 2 inches between each cookie.

8. Bake for 12-15 minutes, or until the edges are lightly browned.

9. Allow the cookies to cool on the baking sheet for 5 minutes before transferring them to a wire rack to cool completely.

Nutritional Information

- Calories: 130
- Fat: 5g
- Carbohydrates: 20g
- Fiber: 2g
- Protein: 2g

CHAPTER SEVEN

Tips for Living with Gastroparesis

Lifestyle Changes That Can Help Manage Symptoms

Gastroparesis is a condition in which the stomach takes longer than normal to empty its contents. This can lead to symptoms such as nausea, vomiting, bloating, and abdominal pain. While there is no cure for gastroparesis, making certain lifestyle changes can help manage symptoms and improve quality of life.

Dietary Modifications

One of the most important lifestyle changes that can help manage symptoms of gastroparesis is modifying your diet. This can include:

1. Eating smaller, more frequent meals: Rather than having three large meals a day, try having six smaller meals to help ease digestion and reduce the workload on your stomach.

2. Chewing your food well: Chewing your food well can help break it down into smaller pieces, making it easier for your stomach to digest.

3. Avoiding high-fat and high-fiber foods: These types of foods can be difficult for your stomach to digest and can worsen symptoms.

4. Drinking plenty of fluids: Staying hydrated can help

prevent constipation and improve digestion. However, it's important to avoid drinking too much at once, as this can cause discomfort and bloating.

Exercise

Regular exercise can also help manage symptoms of gastroparesis. This is because exercise can improve digestion and promote regular bowel movements.

1. Low-impact exercise: Choose low-impact exercises such as walking, yoga, or swimming, as high-impact exercises can worsen symptoms.

2. Light stretching: Gentle stretching can help relieve tension and promote relaxation, which can also help ease symptoms of gastroparesis.

Stress Reduction

Stress can worsen symptoms of gastroparesis, so finding ways to manage stress can be helpful.

1. Mindfulness meditation: Practicing mindfulness meditation can help reduce stress and promote relaxation.

2. Deep breathing exercises: Deep breathing exercises can help calm the nervous system and reduce stress.

3. Yoga: Practicing yoga can help reduce stress and promote relaxation.

Medications

In addition to lifestyle changes, there are medications that can be used to manage symptoms of gastroparesis. These can include:

1. Prokinetic medications: These medications help

improve stomach emptying and can reduce symptoms such as nausea and vomiting.

2. Anti-nausea medications: These medications can be helpful in reducing nausea and vomiting.

3. Pain medications: Pain medications may be prescribed to help manage abdominal pain associated with gastroparesis.

Eating Tips for Managing Gastroparesis

Managing gastroparesis can be challenging, especially when it comes to eating. Here are some eating tips that can help manage symptoms and improve digestion.

Eating Habits

1. Eat small, frequent meals: Rather than having three large meals a day, try having six smaller meals to help ease digestion and reduce the workload on your stomach.

2. Chew your food well: Chewing your food well can help break it down into smaller pieces, making it easier for your stomach to digest.

3. Eat slowly: Eating slowly can help prevent overeating and reduce the workload on your stomach.

4. Avoid drinking fluids with meals: Drinking fluids with meals can cause your stomach to feel overly full and can worsen symptoms.

Food Choices

1. Choose low-fat foods: High-fat foods can be difficult for your stomach to digest and can worsen symptoms. Opt for low-fat foods instead.

2. Choose low-fiber foods: High-fiber foods can be difficult for your stomach to digest and can worsen symptoms.

Choose low-fiber foods such as white bread, pasta, and rice.

3. Avoid carbonated drinks: Carbonated drinks can cause bloating and discomfort, so it's best to avoid them.

4. Limit or avoid alcohol: Alcohol can worsen symptoms of gastroparesis and should be limited or avoided altogether.

5. Avoid spicy or acidic foods: Spicy or acidic foods can irritate the stomach lining and worsen symptoms.

Meal Planning

Meal planning can be helpful in managing gastroparesis. Here are some tips for meal planning:

1. Plan ahead: Plan your meals ahead of time to ensure you have the right foods on hand.

2. Cook in advance: Consider cooking your meals in advance so that you have healthy, easy-to-digest meals ready when you need them.

3. Use smaller plates: Using smaller plates can help you control your portions and prevent overeating.

4. Keep a food diary: Keeping a food diary can help you track your symptoms and identify foods that worsen them.

Coping Strategies for Living with Gastroparesis

Living with gastroparesis can be challenging, both physically and emotionally. Here are some coping strategies that can help you manage the condition and improve your quality of life.

Support

Having a support system can be incredibly helpful when living with gastroparesis. Here are some ways to build a support system:

1. Join a support group: Joining a support group can help you connect with others who are going through similar experiences.

2. Talk to a therapist: Talking to a therapist can help you cope with the emotional challenges of living with gastroparesis.

3. Educate your family and friends: Educating your family and friends about your condition can help them understand what you're going through and how they can support you.

Self-Care

Taking care of yourself is important when living with gastroparesis. Here are some self-care strategies:

1. Get enough rest: Getting enough rest can help you manage symptoms and improve your overall health.

2. Practice relaxation techniques: Practicing relaxation techniques such as deep breathing, meditation, or yoga can help reduce stress and improve your overall well-being.

3. Stay active: Regular exercise can help improve digestion and promote regular bowel movements.

4. Take time for yourself: Taking time for yourself to do things you enjoy can help you cope with the emotional challenges of living with gastroparesis.

Coping with Symptoms

Managing symptoms of gastroparesis can be challenging. Here are some coping strategies:

1. Keep a symptom diary: Keeping a symptom diary can help you track your symptoms and identify triggers.

2. Use heat or cold therapy: Applying heat or cold therapy to your abdomen can help relieve pain and discomfort.

3. Try over-the-counter remedies: Over-the-counter remedies such as ginger, peppermint, or chamomile tea can help relieve nausea and other symptoms.

4. Work with your doctor: Working with your doctor to find the right treatment plan can help you manage symptoms and improve your quality of life.

Living with gastroparesis can be challenging, but making certain lifestyle changes and implementing coping strategies can help manage symptoms and improve quality of life. Remember to seek support from family, friends, and healthcare professionals to help you cope with the emotional challenges of the condition.

CONCLUSION

The Importance of the Gastroparesis Diet

Gastroparesis is a digestive disorder that affects the stomach's ability to move food through the digestive system. It can cause a range of symptoms, including nausea, vomiting, and abdominal pain. While there is no cure for gastroparesis, following a gastroparesis diet can help manage the symptoms and improve overall digestive health.

The gastroparesis diet involves eating foods that are easy to digest and move through the digestive system, such as low-fat and low-fiber foods. Some of the main principles of the gastroparesis diet include eating small, frequent meals, avoiding fatty and greasy foods, and limiting the intake of fiber and raw fruits and vegetables.

One of the primary goals of the gastroparesis diet is to help the stomach empty more efficiently. Eating smaller, more frequent meals can help prevent the stomach from becoming too full and overloading the digestive system. Avoiding fatty and greasy foods can also help since they can slow down digestion and make it harder for the stomach to empty.

Another key component of the gastroparesis diet is limiting the intake of fiber. Fiber can be difficult for the stomach to digest, especially when it is not functioning properly. Raw fruits and vegetables, in particular, can be hard to digest, so it is recommended to cook them before eating to make them easier on the stomach.

Overall, the gastroparesis diet is an important part of managing gastroparesis symptoms and improving digestive health. While it may require some adjustments to your eating habits, following the guidelines can help alleviate symptoms and improve quality of life.

How the Cookbook Can Help Those with Gastroparesis

Following a gastroparesis diet can be challenging, especially for those who enjoy cooking and trying new foods. However, with the right resources, it is possible to eat delicious and satisfying meals while still adhering to the diet. This is where the gastroparesis cookbook can be incredibly helpful.

The gastroparesis cookbook is a collection of recipes specifically designed for those with gastroparesis. The recipes are tailored to be low in fat and fiber and easy to digest, making them ideal for those with digestive issues. The cookbook also includes tips for meal planning and preparation, as well as suggestions for modifying recipes to fit individual dietary needs.

One of the benefits of using the gastroparesis cookbook is that it takes the guesswork out of meal planning. With a range of recipes to choose from, it is easier to plan meals that are both nutritious and satisfying. Plus, since the recipes are designed specifically for those with gastroparesis, they take into account the unique dietary needs of the condition.

Another benefit of using the gastroparesis cookbook is that it can help broaden your culinary horizons. Following a restricted diet can be frustrating and limiting, but the cookbook offers a wide range of recipes to try. From soups and stews to baked goods and desserts, there are plenty of options to choose from. This can help prevent boredom and make it easier to stick to the diet long-term.

In conclusion, the gastroparesis diet and cookbook are important resources for those with gastroparesis. Following the guidelines of the diet can help manage symptoms and improve digestive health, while the cookbook can make it easier and more enjoyable to stick to the diet long-term. By working with a healthcare provider and utilizing these resources, those with gastroparesis can improve their quality of life and enjoy delicious, satisfying meals.

Appendix

List of resources for further reading

1. Google Scholar: A search engine for scholarly literature, including articles, theses, books, and conference papers.

2. ResearchGate: A social networking site for scientists and researchers to share papers, ask and answer questions, and find collaborators.

3. arXiv: An open-access repository for scholarly articles in physics, mathematics, computer science, and other scientific disciplines.

4. PubMed: A free database of biomedical literature, including articles and research papers.

5. JSTOR: A digital library of academic journals, books, and primary sources in various subjects, including history, art, and economics.

www.ingramcontent.com/pod-product-compliance
Lightning Source LLC
Chambersburg PA
CBHW050927260726
48660CB00001B/432